FREEDOM FROM INFERTILITY IN WOMEN

Daily Affirmations that will make you fruitful.

BY
IHEKE WILLIAMS

Unless otherwise indicated, all scripture quotations are taken from the King James Version of the Bible A key for other Bible versions used;

NKJV	New King James Version
AMP	The Amplified Bible
TANT	The New Amplified Bible
TLB -	The Living Bible
CEV -	Contemporary English Version
NASB	New American Standard Version
GW -	God's Word version
ESV -	English Standard Version
NET -	New English Translation
ISV -	International Standard Version
NIV -	New International Version
MSG -	The Message Translation

DEDICATION

This Book is dedicated to Almighty God and to every married couple in the world.

TABLE OF CONTENT

WHAT IS INFERTILITY?

Infertility is "a disease of the reproductive system defined by the failure to achieve a clinical pregnancy after 12 months or more of regular unprotected sexual intercourse (and there is no other reason, such as breastfeeding or postpartum amenorrhea).

Primary infertility is infertility in a couple who have never had a child. Secondary infertility is failure to conceive following a previous pregnancy. Infertility may be caused by infection in the man or woman, but often there is no obvious underlying cause.

Source: WHO, Wikipedia

WHAT IS GOD'S SOLUTION

But He was wounded for our transgressions, he was bruised for our iniquities: the chastisement of our peace was upon Him; and with His stripes we are healed – Isaiah 53:5 (KJV)

"...By His wounds ye have been healed" – 1 Peter 2:24 (KJV)

The phrase "...ye **HAVE BEEN HEALED**" is in the past tense, it means that JESUS has ALREADY HEALED your reproductive organs including your womb and, the reproductive organs of your husband as well, years ago.

You have NO business with barrenness. You are Fruitful.

You are Healed already, productive and active Forever. There is Divine Health in you and in your husband because of what Jesus did for you on the cross.

For the next 31 days and forever, you will affirm this blessing that Our Lord Jesus Christ has given to you and you will you live in perfect health FOREVER!.

INSTRUCTION 1

That if thou shalt <u>confess with thy mouth</u> the Lord Jesus, and shalt <u>believe in thine heart</u> that God hath raised him from the dead, thou shalt be saved. – Romans 10:9

We having the same <u>spirit of faith</u>, according as it is written, I believed, and therefore have I spoken; <u>we also believe, and therefore speak</u>; - 2 Corinthians 4:13

There has to be a connection with what you say/affirm with your mouth and what you have in your heart or what you believe in your heart.

Consequently, for the affirmations to be effective, you will have to meditate on the scripture (1 Peter 2:24) for 5 minutes, in your heart, before you affirm it with your mouth.

Don't say anything to the contrary during the period of affirmations.

INSTRUCTION 2

"...By His wounds ye have been healed" –
1 Peter 2:24 (KJV)

Divine Health is inside you whether or not you believe it. You might not feel or see it, but it is in you already. As you affirm it that you have been healed, it will be activated to do it's work.

For the duration of the affirmations, always place your hands on your stomach as you affirm the blessings.

Affirm this Blessings consistently each day.

Follow these instructions, **BE CONSISTENT** and your affirmations will be very effective.

DAY 1
AFFIRMATION

Meditate on 1 Peter 2:24B for 5 minutes

"···By His Stripes ye have been healed"

Place your hands on your stomach and affirm the blessing

"I HAVE BEEN HEALED THEREFORE I AFFIRM THAT MY WOMB IS ACTIVE AND FRUITFUL"

DAY 2
AFFIRMATION

Meditate on 1 Peter 2:24B for 5 minutes

"⋯By His Stripes ye have been healed"

Place your hands on your stomach and affirm the blessing

"I HAVE BEEN HEALED THEREFORE I AFFIRM THAT MY WOMB IS ACTIVE AND PRODUCTIVE"

DAY 3
AFFIRMATION

Meditate on 1 Peter 2:24B for 5 minutes

" ···By His Stripes ye have been healed"

<u>Place your hands on your stomach and affirm the blessing</u>

"I HAVE BEEN HEALED THEREFORE I AFFIRM THAT MY REPRODUCTIVE ORGANS ARE ACTIVE AND FRUITFUL "

DAY 4
AFFIRMATION

Meditate on 1 Peter 2:24B for 5 minutes

"···By His Stripes ye have been healed"

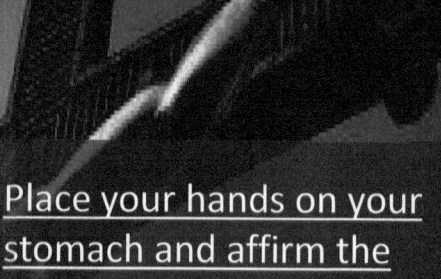

Place your hands on your stomach and affirm the blessing

"I HAVE BEEN HEALED THEREFORE I AFFIRM THAT MY OVULATION IS ACTIVE AND NORMAL"

DAY 5
AFFIRMATION

Meditate on 1 Peter
2:24B for 5 minutes

"···By His
Stripes ye have
been healed"

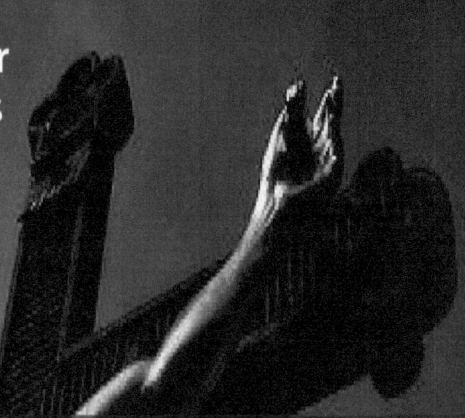

Place your hands on your
stomach and affirm the
blessing

"I HAVE BEEN
HEALED
THEREFORE
I AFFIRM THAT MY
OVARIES ARE
ACTIVE AND
FRUITFUL"

DAY 6
AFFIRMATION

Meditate on 1 Peter 2:24B for 5 minutes

"…By His Stripes ye have been healed"

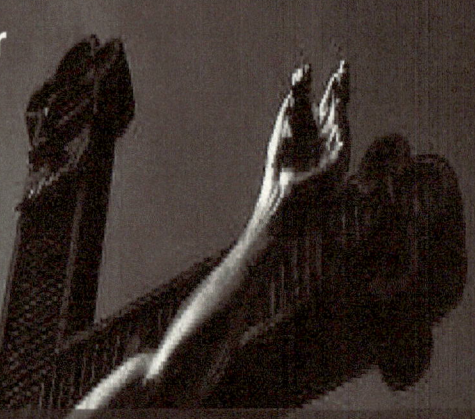

Place your hands on your stomach and affirm the blessing

*"*I HAVE BEEN HEALED THEREFORE I AFFIRM THAT MY HORMONES ARE ACTIVE, NORMAL, BALANCED AND FRUITFUL *"*

DAY 7
AFFIRMATION

Meditate on 1 Peter 2:24B for 5 minutes

"···By His Stripes ye have been healed"

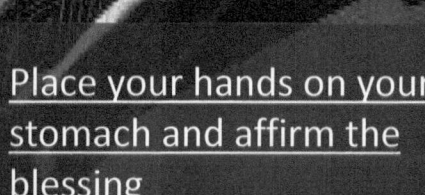

Place your hands on your stomach and affirm the blessing

"I HAVE BEEN HEALED THEREFORE I AFFIRM THAT MY EGGS ARE ACTIVE, FERTILE AND FRUITFUL"

DAY 8
AFFIRMATION

Meditate on 1 Peter 2:24B for 5 minutes

"...By His Stripes ye have been healed"

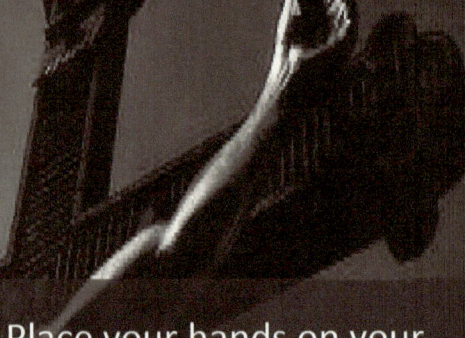

Place your hands on your stomach and affirm the blessing

"I HAVE BEEN HEALED THEREFORE I AFFIRM THAT MY FALOPIAN TUBE IS ACTIVE AND FRUITFUL "

DAY 9
AFFIRMATION

Meditate on 1 Peter 2:24B for 5 minutes

"···By His Stripes ye have been healed"

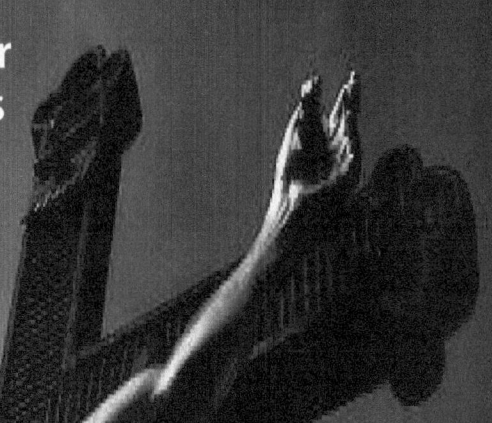

Place your hands on your stomach and affirm the blessing

"I HAVE BEEN HEALED THEREFORE I AFFIRM THAT I HAVE NO SEXUALLY TRANSMITTED INFECTIONS INSIDE ME"

DAY 10
AFFIRMATION

Meditate on 1 Peter
2:24B for 5 minutes

"···By His
Stripes ye have
been healed"

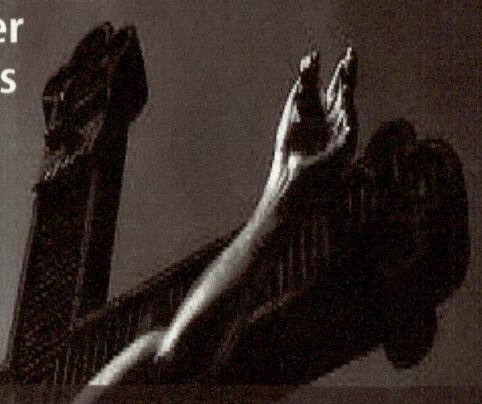

Place your hands on your
stomach and affirm the
blessing

"I HAVE BEEN
HEALED
THEREFORE
I AFFIRM THAT
I AM
ACTIVE AND
FRUITFUL"

DAY 11
AFFIRMATION

Meditate on 1 Peter
2:24B for 5 minutes

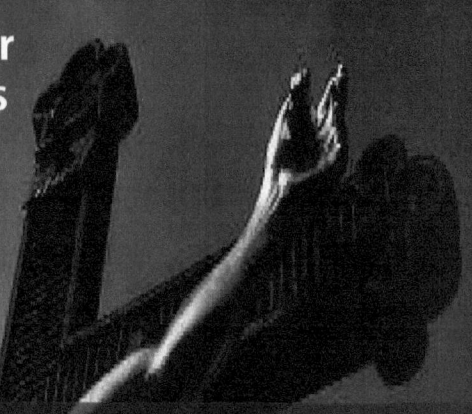

"···By His
Stripes ye have
been healed"

Place your hands on your
stomach and affirm the
blessing

"I HAVE BEEN
HEALED
THEREFORE
I AFFIRM THAT MY
IMMUNE SYSTEM IS
ACTIVE AND
STRONG FOREVER"

DAY 12
AFFIRMATION

Meditate on 1 Peter 2:24B for 5 minutes

"…By His Stripes ye have been healed"

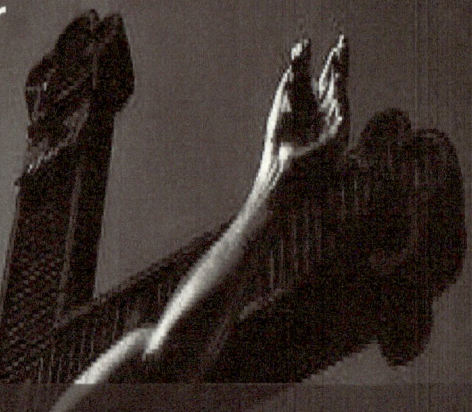

Place your hands on your stomach and affirm the blessing

"I HAVE BEEN HEALED THEREFORE I AFFIRM THAT MY UTERINE CONDITION IS PERFECT AND NORMAL"

DAY 13
AFFIRMATION

Meditate on 1 Peter
2:24B for 5 minutes

"···By His
Stripes ye have
been healed"

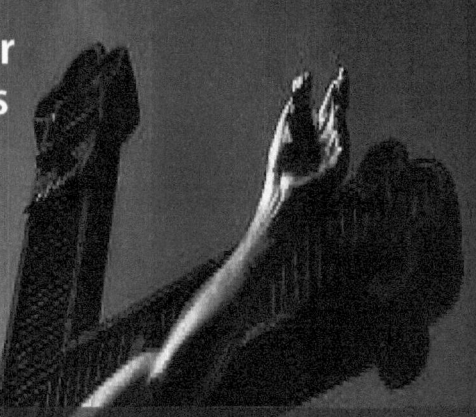

Place your hands on your
stomach and affirm the
blessing

"I HAVE BEEN
HEALED
THEREFORE
I AFFIRM THAT
I DO NOT HAVE
ANY GENETIC
PROBLEMS"

DAY 14
AFFIRMATION

Meditate on 1 Peter
2:24B for 5 minutes

"···By His
Stripes ye have
been healed"

Place your hands on your
stomach and affirm the
blessing

"I HAVE BEEN
HEALED
THEREFORE
I AFFIRM THAT
MY WOMB IS
FRUITFUL"

DAY 15
AFFIRMATION

Meditate on 1 Peter 2:24B for 5 minutes

"…By His Stripes ye have been healed"

Place your hands on your stomach and affirm the blessing

"I HAVE BEEN HEALED THEREFORE I AFFIRM THAT I AM FERTILE"

DAY 16
AFFIRMATION

Meditate on 1 Peter 2:24B for 5 minutes

"···By His Stripes ye have been healed"

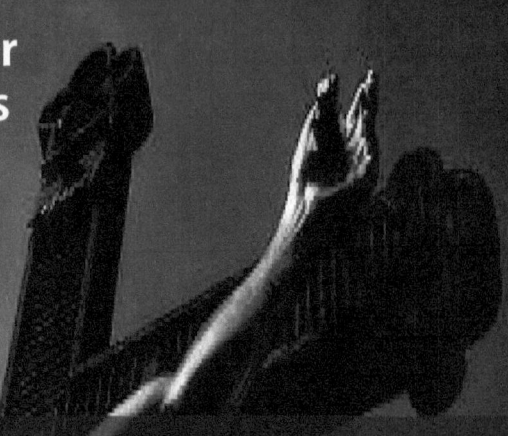

Place your hands on your stomach and affirm the blessing

"MY HUSBAND HAS BEEN HEALED THEREFORE I AFFIRM THAT HIS REPRODUCTIVE ORGANS ARE ACTIVE AND FRUITFUL"

DAY 17
AFFIRMATION

Meditate on 1 Peter 2:24B for 5 minutes

"···By His Stripes ye have been healed"

<u>Place your hands on your stomach and affirm the blessing</u>

"I HAVE BEEN HEALED THEREFORE I AFFIRM THAT MY WOMB IS FRUITFUL"

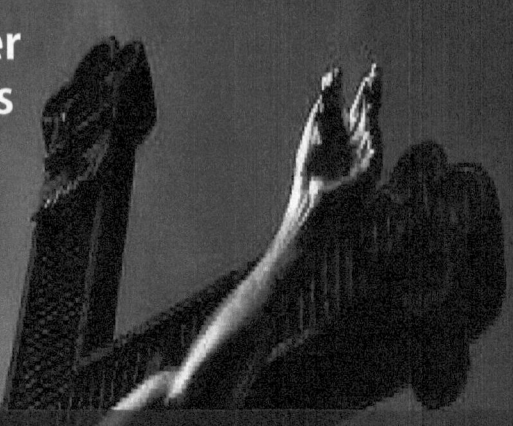

DAY 18
AFFIRMATION

Meditate on 1 Peter 2:24B for 5 minutes

"···By His Stripes ye have been healed"

Place your hands on your stomach and affirm the blessing

"MY HUSBAND HAS BEEN HEALED THEREFORE I AFFIRM THAT HIS REPRODUCTIVE ORGANS ARE ACTIVE AND FRUITFUL"

DAY 19
AFFIRMATION

Meditate on 1 Peter
2:24B for 5 minutes

"···By His
Stripes ye have
been healed"

Place your hands on your
stomach and affirm the
blessing

"I HAVE BEEN
HEALED
THEREFORE
I AFFIRM THAT
MY WOMB IS
FRUITFUL"

DAY 20
AFFIRMATION

Meditate on 1 Peter 2:24B for 5 minutes

"···By His Stripes ye have been healed"

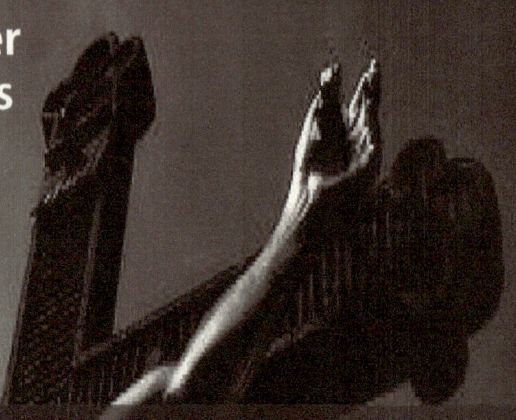

Place your hands on your stomach and affirm the blessing

"MY HUSBAND HAS BEEN HEALED THEREFORE I AFFIRM THAT HIS REPRODUCTIVE ORGANS ARE ACTIVE AND FRUITFUL"

DAY 21
AFFIRMATION

Meditate on 1 Peter 2:24B for 5 minutes

"...By His Stripes ye have been healed"

Place your hands on your stomach and affirm the blessing

"I HAVE BEEN HEALED THEREFORE I AFFIRM THAT MY WOMB IS FRUITFUL"

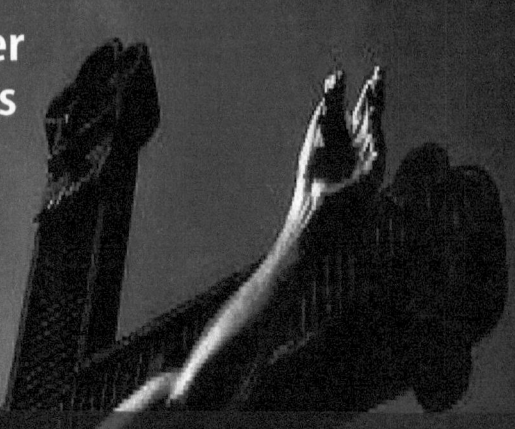

DAY 22
AFFIRMATION

Meditate on 1 Peter 2:24B for 5 minutes

"···By His Stripes ye have been healed"

Place your hands on your stomach and affirm the blessing

"MY HUSBAND HAS BEEN HEALED THEREFORE I AFFIRM THAT HIS REPRODUCTIVE ORGANS ARE ACTIVE AND FRUITFUL"

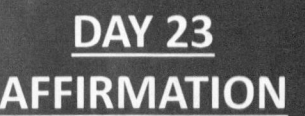

DAY 23
AFFIRMATION

Meditate on 1 Peter
2:24B for 5 minutes

"···By His
Stripes ye have
been healed"

Place your hands on your
stomach and affirm the
blessing

"I HAVE BEEN
HEALED
THEREFORE
I AFFIRM THAT
MY WOMB IS
FRUITFUL"

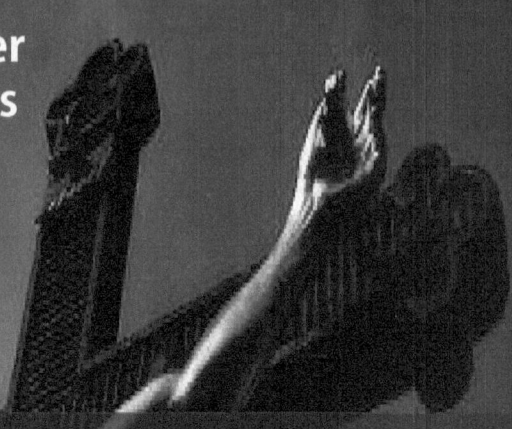

DAY 24
AFFIRMATION

Meditate on 1 Peter 2:24B for 5 minutes

"...By His Stripes ye have been healed"

Place your hands on your stomach and affirm the blessing

"MY HUSBAND HAS BEEN HEALED THEREFORE I AFFIRM THAT HIS REPRODUCTIVE ORGANS ARE ACTIVE AND FRUITFUL"

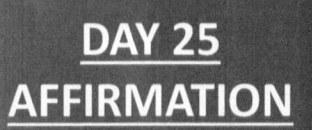

DAY 25
AFFIRMATION

Meditate on 1 Peter 2:24B for 5 minutes

"...By His Stripes ye have been healed"

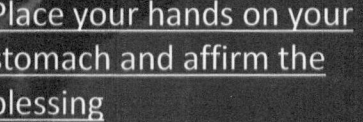

Place your hands on your stomach and affirm the blessing

"I HAVE BEEN HEALED THEREFORE I AFFIRM THAT MY WOMB IS FRUITFUL"

DAY 26
AFFIRMATION

Meditate on 1 Peter 2:24B for 5 minutes

"...By His Stripes ye have been healed"

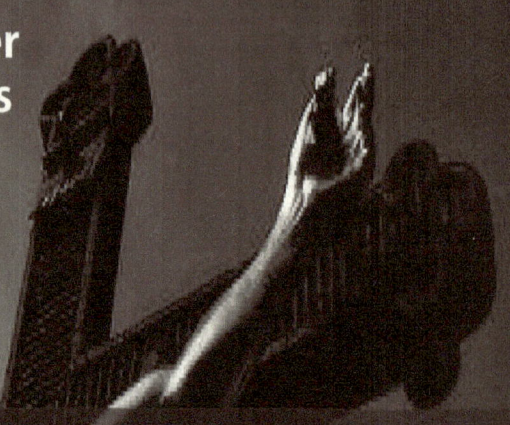

Place your hands on your stomach and affirm the blessing

"MY HUSBAND HAS BEEN HEALED THEREFORE I AFFIRM THAT HIS REPRODUCTIVE ORGANS ARE ACTIVE AND FRUITFUL"

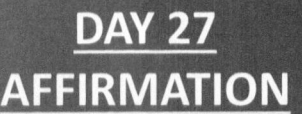

DAY 27
AFFIRMATION

Meditate on 1 Peter 2:24B for 5 minutes

"···By His Stripes ye have been healed"

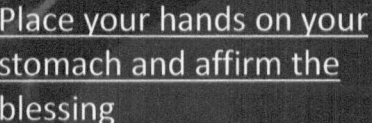

Place your hands on your stomach and affirm the blessing

"I HAVE BEEN HEALED THEREFORE I AFFIRM THAT MY WOMB IS FRUITFUL"

DAY 28
AFFIRMATION

Meditate on 1 Peter 2:24B for 5 minutes

"···By His Stripes ye have been healed"

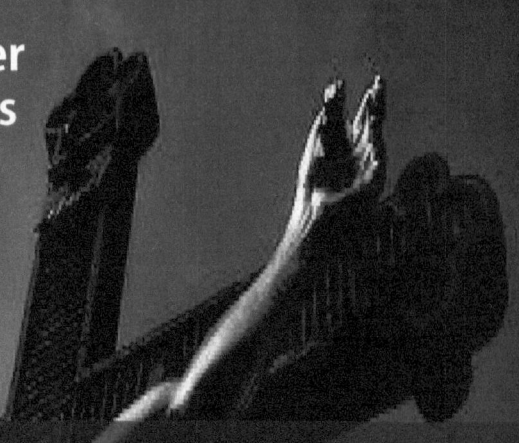

Place your hands on your stomach and affirm the blessing

"MY HUSBAND HAS BEEN HEALED THEREFORE I AFFIRM THAT HIS REPRODUCTIVE ORGANS ARE ACTIVE AND FRUITFUL"

DAY 29
AFFIRMATION

Meditate on 1 Peter 2:24B for 5 minutes

"···By His Stripes ye have been healed"

Place your hands on your stomach and affirm the blessing

"I HAVE BEEN HEALED THEREFORE I AFFIRM THAT MY WOMB IS FRUITFUL"

DAY 30
AFFIRMATION

Meditate on 1 Peter
2:24B for 5 minutes

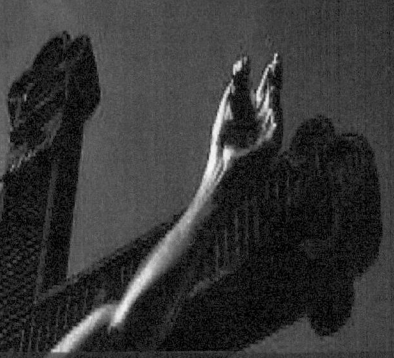

"···By His
Stripes ye have
been healed"

Place your hands on your
stomach and affirm the
blessing

"I HAVE BEEN
HEALED
THEREFORE
I AFFIRM THAT
MY WOMB IS
FRUITFUL"

DAY 31
AFFIRMATION

Meditate on 1 Peter 2:24B for 5 minutes

"···By His Stripes ye have been healed"

Place your hands on your stomach and affirm the blessing

"I HAVE BEEN HEALED THEREFORE I AFFIRM THAT MY WOMB IS FRUITFUL"

"..by His stripes ye HAVE BEEN HEALED"- 1 PETER 2:24

Jesus Christ has paid the price for your peace. Don't let Satan deceive you that you are barren.

Don't let Satan put you in bondage any longer.

Your body has been healed already. You have NO business with infertility.

You and your husband are ACTIVE, STRONG and FRUITFUL FOREVER!

You are FREE from sickness FOREVER because of what Jesus did for you on the cross.

PRAYER FOR SALVATION

We believe that you have been blessed and that you want to receive eternal life that God has made available to everyone who believes in his love and his grace which He expressed lavishly through His Son Jesus Christ.

"For God so loved the world, that He gave his only begotten Son, that whosoever believeth in him should not perish, but have everlasting life." - John 3:16

Say this prayer to God and believe it with your heart

"Father, I believe that you gave me your only Son to die for my sin. I believe you raised Him from the dead. I declare that your son, Jesus Christ is the Lord of my life. I receive eternal life and I receive the Holy Spirit. I am saved forever.in Jesus name. I am so Happy that today and forever, I am your child. Amen ".

Congratulations, you are now a child of God Halleluyah!! – John 1:12

OTHER INFORMATION

Please share your testimonies via the following handles;

ihekewilliams@gmail.com
+2348061530541

Other Books written by the author includes

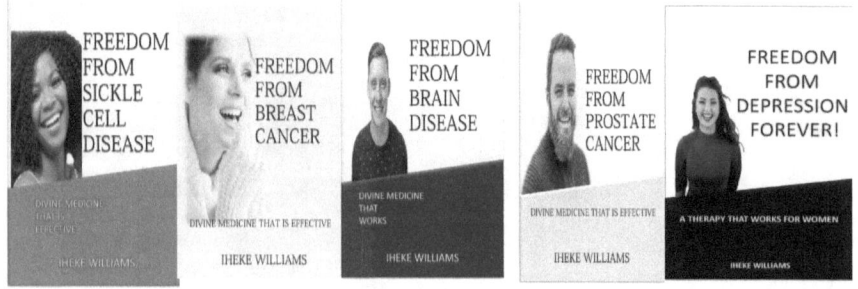

Visit us on Amazon by clicking on the link below;

https://www.amazon.com/Iheke-w.-Okpara/e/B01KFYO1PU/ref=ntt_dp_epwbk_0

ABOUT THE AUTHOR

Iheke Williams is a firm follower and disciple of the Lord Jesus Christ. He is a passionate minister of the grace of our Lord and savior Jesus Christ and has brought the reality of the divine life of Christ into the lives of so many.

Iheke Williams has a calling to communicate the gospel of Christ with simplicity and to show the world how to activate the eternal life of God that is in us already which includes Divine health, Divine righteousness, Divine security and Divine prosperity.

As you read this book and other books written by Iheke Williams you will literally begin to function and manifest the life of God that is already inside you to the glory of God the Father who is the author of all grace and mercy. Amen.

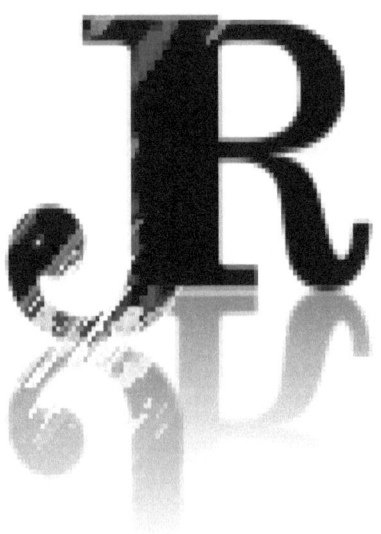

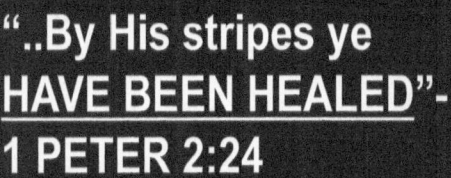

"..By His stripes ye
<u>HAVE BEEN HEALED</u>"-
1 PETER 2:24

YOU
ARE
FREE
FOREVER!!

FREEDOM SERIES

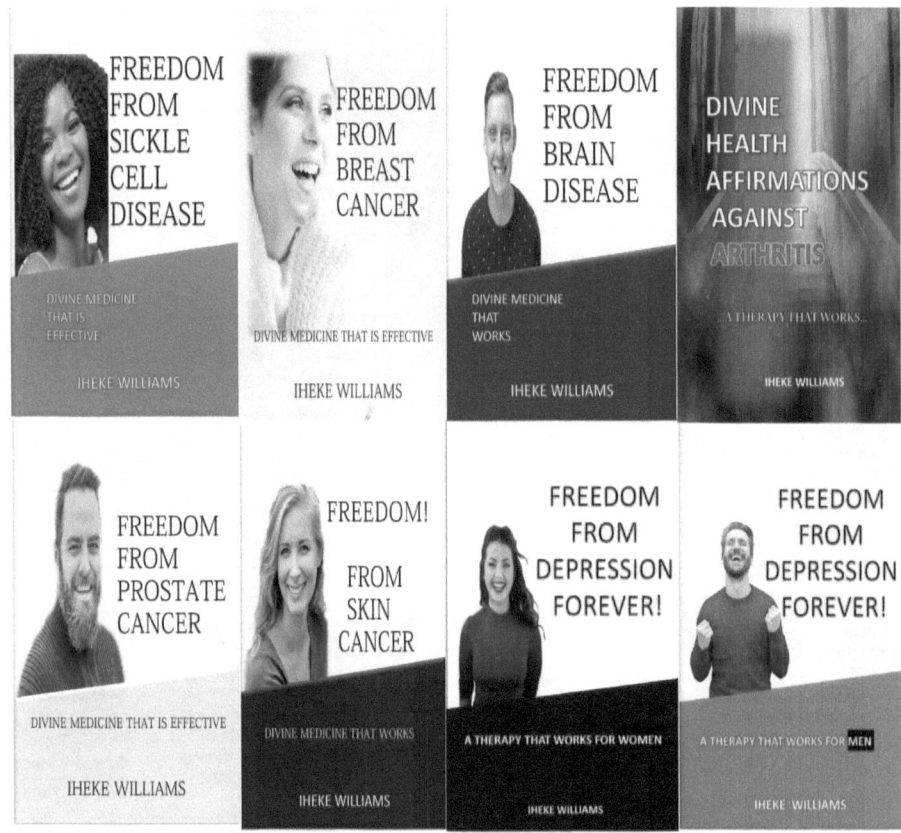

https://www.amazon.com/Iheke-w.-Okpara/e/B01KFYO1PU/ref=ntt_dp_epwbk_0